Flurina Christina Clement
Ramiro Dip
Hanspeter Naegeli

Glycidamide-induced expression signature

Flurina Christina Clement
Ramiro Dip
Hanspeter Naegeli

Glycidamide-induced expression signature

Transcriptional fingerprint of glycidamide,
the reactive metabolite of the widespread
food carcinogen acrylamide

Südwestdeutscher Verlag für Hochschulschriften

Impressum/Imprint (nur für Deutschland/ only for Germany)
Bibliografische Information der Deutschen Nationalbibliothek: Die Deutsche Nationalbibliothek verzeichnet diese Publikation in der Deutschen Nationalbibliografie; detaillierte bibliografische Daten sind im Internet über http://dnb.d-nb.de abrufbar.
Alle in diesem Buch genannten Marken und Produktnamen unterliegen warenzeichen-, markenoder patentrechtlichem Schutz bzw. sind Warenzeichen oder eingetragene Warenzeichen der jeweiligen Inhaber. Die Wiedergabe von Marken, Produktnamen, Gebrauchsnamen, Handelsnamen, Warenbezeichnungen u.s.w. in diesem Werk berechtigt auch ohne besondere Kennzeichnung nicht zu der Annahme, dass solche Namen im Sinne der Warenzeichen- und Markenschutzgesetzgebung als frei zu betrachten wären und daher von jedermann benutzt werden dürften.

Verlag: Südwestdeutscher Verlag für Hochschulschriften Aktiengesellschaft & Co. KG
Dudweiler Landstr. 99, 66123 Saarbrücken, Deutschland
Telefon +49 681 37 20 271-1, Telefax +49 681 37 20 271-0, Email: info@svh-verlag.de
Zugl.: Zurich, University of Zurich, Diss., 2007

Herstellung in Deutschland:
Schaltungsdienst Lange o.H.G., Berlin
Books on Demand GmbH, Norderstedt
Reha GmbH, Saarbrücken
Amazon Distribution GmbH, Leipzig
ISBN: 978-3-8381-0630-4

Imprint (only for USA, GB)
Bibliographic information published by the Deutsche Nationalbibliothek: The Deutsche Nationalbibliothek lists this publication in the Deutsche Nationalbibliografie; detailed bibliographic data are available in the Internet at http://dnb.d-nb.de.
Any brand names and product names mentioned in this book are subject to trademark, brand or patent protection and are trademarks or registered trademarks of their respective holders. The use of brand names, product names, common names, trade names, product descriptions etc. even without a particular marking in this works is in no way to be construed to mean that such names may be regarded as unrestricted in respect of trademark and brand protection legislation and could thus be used by anyone.

Publisher:
Südwestdeutscher Verlag für Hochschulschriften Aktiengesellschaft & Co. KG
Dudweiler Landstr. 99, 66123 Saarbrücken, Germany
Phone +49 681 37 20 271-1, Fax +49 681 37 20 271-0, Email: info@svh-verlag.de

Copyright © 2009 by the author and Südwestdeutscher Verlag für Hochschulschriften Aktiengesellschaft & Co. KG and licensors
All rights reserved. Saarbrücken 2009

Printed in the U.S.A.
Printed in the U.K. by (see last page)
ISBN: 978-3-8381-0630-4

TABLE OF CONTENTS

1.	SUMMARY	3
2.	INTRODUCTION	4
2.1.	The HEATOX project	4
2.2.	Acrylamide and its formation in food	4
2.3.	Glycidamide and detoxification processes	5
2.4.	Carcinogenesis	6
2.5.	Biomarkers	7
2.6.	Basic principle	8
2.7.	Aims	9
3.	MATERIALS AND METHODS	10
3.1.	Chemicals	10
3.2.	Cell culture and treatments	10
3.3.	Cytotoxicity and caspase assays	11
3.4.	Gene expression analysis	11
3.5.	Real-time quantitative RT-PCR	12
3.6.	Glutathione assay	12
3.7.	NF-κB reporter assay	13
4.	RESULTS	14
4.1.	Glycidamide toxicity	14
4.2.	Expression profiling	15
4.3.	Multivariate analysis of transcriptomes	17
4.4.	Univariate transcriptome analysis	18
4.5.	Data verification by RT-PCR analysis	24
4.6.	Changes of GSH status	27

4.7.	NF-κB activation	30
5.	DISCUSSION	32
6.	SIGNIFICANCE	38
7.	REFERENCES	40

compound is generated in many common foods during cooking at high temperatures (Svensson et al. 2003). For example, acrylamide reaches parts per million concentrations in French fries, potato and tortilla chips, bread crust, various baked goods, breakfast cereals and coffee.

It was soon recognized that acrylamide is formed during the Maillard browning reaction from a heat-induced reaction between the amino acid asparagine and the carbonyl group of glucose (Mottram et al. 2002; Stadler et al. 2002). The Maillard browning is a non-enzymatic reaction, firstly described by Louis Maillard in 1912. It is characterized by the condensation of an amino group with a reducing sugar moiety when temperatures of more than 120°C are applied at conditions that reduce the local water content. The Maillard reaction is responsible for the typical taste, appearance and texture of the affected food items. Thus, most of the effects of this reaction, such as the introduction of caramel aromas and the golden brown color, are desirable. Unwanted effects of the Maillard reaction include the excessive food darkening, the off-flavor development and the generation of acrylamide.

2.3. *Glycidamide and detoxification processes*

A large fraction of the ingested acrylamide is converted to glycidamide by a member of the cytochrome P-450 superfamily, i.e., by cytochrome P-450 2E1 (CYP2E1) monooxygenase (Fig. 1). Glycidamide is an epoxide derivative that is substantially more reactive towards cellular macromolecules than acrylamide itself (Sumner et al. 1999). Unlike acrylamide, glycidamide has been found to yield positive results in the Ames test performed with *Salmonella* strains, implying that it displays a mutagenic activity (Hashimoto and Tanii 1985). In mammalian and human cells, glycidamide generates DNA strand breaks and induced the formation of different kinds of base adducts (Gamboa da Costa et al. 2003; Besaratinia and Pfeiffer 2003; Doerge et al. 2005), and these hazardous DNA lesions may be responsible for the mutagenic properties of glycidamide (Besaratinia and Pfeiffer 2004). When tested with short-term rodent studies, glycidamide generates micronuclei in white blood cells, thus confirming that this compound displays potentially deleterious DNA-damaging effects (Paulsson et al. 2003; Baum et al. 2005; Puppel et al. 2005; Manjanatha et al. 2006).

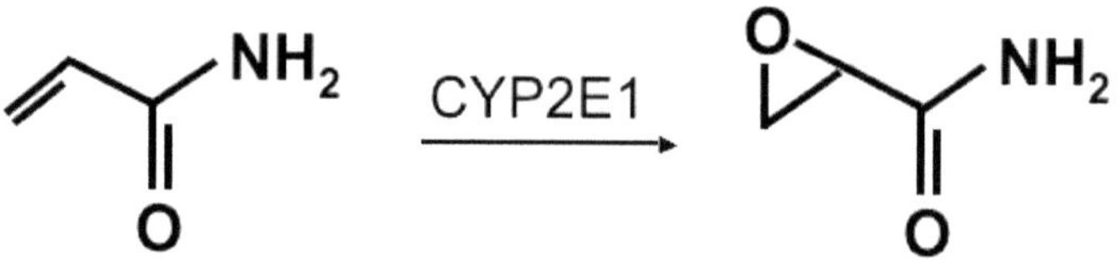

Figure 1. Molecular structure of acrylamide and glycidamide. Acrylamide is converted into glycidamide by cytochrome P-450 2E1 (CYP2E1).

Both acrylamide and glycidamide are rapidly detoxified by the action of glutathione-S-transferase, which catalyzes the conjugation with glutathione (GSH). Subsequently, the resulting GSH conjugates are converted to mercapturic acid metabolites that are excreted in the urine. In addition, glycidamide is additionally inactivated by cleavage of the epoxide ring through the action of epoxide hydrolases (Odlund et al. 1994; Tong et al. 2004).

2.4. Carcinogenesis

The long-term carcinogenicity studies in mice and rats demonstrated tumor induction by acrylamide at daily doses of 1 mg/kg body weight or higher (Friedman et al. 1995). This apparent threshold for tumor induction in rodents exceeds the ordinary dietary exposure of humans by several orders of magnitude. In fact, the average dietary intake of acrylamide in Western populations has been estimated to be in the range of ~0.5 µg/kg body weight/day (Konings et al. 2003; Svensson et al. 2003; Dybing et al. 2005), although children may be more highly exposed. Occupational exposures have been estimated in the daily range of 1 µg/kg body weight, whereas cigarette smoking leads to a considerably higher acrylamide intake of ~3 µg/kg/day (Bergmark 1997). Based on the rodent studies, conventional low-dose extrapolations have been made for the incidence of human cancer associated with the ingestion of acrylamide contained in foods or beverages. Different quantitative estimates of lifetime cancer risks in human population range from 1 per 10'000 to 4.4 per 1'000 exposed individuals (reviewed by Dybing and Sanner 2003). On the other hand, exposure to acrylamide could not be linked to increased cancer mortality in any epidemiologic study (Marsh et al. 1999; Mucci et al. 2003; Rice 2005; Pelucchi et al. 2006). Therefore, it remains difficult to establish the full extent of health risks resulting from the wide appearance of this food carcinogen (Erdreich and Friedman 2004).

2.5. Biomarkers

Because of their short half-lives, the detection of acrylamide or glycidamide in the blood or tissue of exposed people has remained elusive. However, hemoglobin adducts in blood, mercapturic acid metabolites in the urine or DNA adducts in target tissues have been proposed as indirect biomarkers to assess the internal exposure to acrylamide and its genotoxic metabolite glycidamide (Calleman et al. 1994; Bergmark 1997; Manière et al. 2005; Fuhr et al. 2006). This approach has been useful for example to estimate the level of glycidamide that arises transiently in human blood after the consumption of acrylamide-containing food (unpublished results from the HEATOX consortium). On the other hand, it is not clear what level of hemoglobin adducts, urine metabolites, DNA adducts or other kinds of molecular damage could be tolerated without exceeding an acceptable level of cancer risk. As a consequence, we have performed a large-scale transcriptomic analysis, using high-density DNA microarrays, to identify differentially expressed genes that may be used as a true biomarker of hazardous effects in exposed tissues.

2.6. Basic principle

Traditional approaches in toxicology involve the use of high doses of the chemicals under scrutiny, thus inducing some kind of severe damage to organs, tissues, cells, organelles or macromolecules. Alternatively, a large number of cellular bioassays have been developed to assess molecular responses to potentially toxic compounds. In most cases, the tested chemical is able to stimulate a particular receptor, leading to activation of signaling cascades that eventually induce an active cellular response such as apoptosis, gene induction, protein modification or other biochemical reactions.

Traditional bioassays are normally focused on the measurement of a single cellular response. However, a new approach in toxicology takes advantage of newly developed large-scale analyses such as transcriptomics or proteomics. Using these large-scale strategies it has become possible to monitor multiple endpoints simultaneously, thus obtaining molecular profiles or "fingerprints" that are characteristic for the action of particular groups of toxic chemicals (Fig. 2). Transcriptomics is based on the simultaneous quantitative measurement of a large number of messenger RNA transcripts coding for specific cellular proteins.

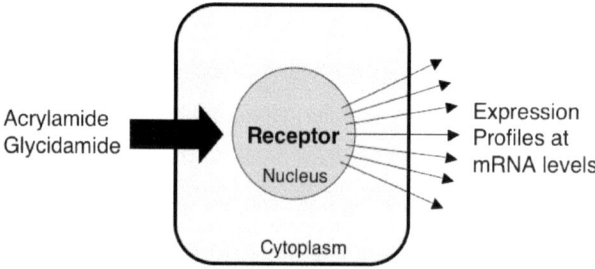

Figure 2: *Principle of multi-endpoint bioassays enabling expression profiles monitoring at mRNA levels.*

A standard human breast tumor cell line (MCF7) was selected as the primary target of these transcriptomic experiments because the lifetime rodent studies yielded mammary gland adenomas and adenocarcinomas in females (Friedman et al. 1995), and because the appearance of acrylamide in mammary glands has been demonstrated after ingestion of contaminated food (Sorgel et al. 2002). The selected MCF7 cells have been shown to display intact p53-dependent reactions, including cell cycle arrest and apoptosis, in response to DNA damaging agents (Calcabrini et al. 2006; Hernandez-Vargas et al. 2006; Ray et al. 2006). Additionally, the human colonic cell line CaCo-2 has been tested as a system that mimics the absorptive barrier of an intestinal epithelium (Meunier et al. 1995).

2.7. Aims

The goal of the present study was to use the most advanced transcriptomic platform to monitor, at the transcriptional level, the expression changes induced in human cells by exposure to acrylamide or glycidamide. The purpose of these studies was to test whether the genomic reprogramming elicited by acrylamide or glycidamide may potentiate or, alternatively, counteract the known genotoxic effects of these compounds.

3. MATERIALS AND METHODS

3.1. Chemicals

Glycidamide was purchased from Toronto Research Chemicals (Canada) and acrylamide was from Fluka (Buchs, Switzerland). Both chemicals were dissolved in distilled water. All other reagents used were of the highest purity that is commercially available.

3.2. Cell culture and treatments

All cell culture media were from Gibco. The MCF7 cell line subtype BUS (provided by A. M. Soto and C. Sonnenschein, Tufts University, Boston, USA) was grown in Dulbecco's Modified Eagle Medium (DMEM) supplemented with 10% fetal bovine serum (FBS). The antibiotics used were 0.1 U/ml penicillin and 0.1 µg/ml streptomycin. CaCo-2 cells (obtained from A. Pospischil, Institute of Veterinary Pathology, University of Zürich, Switzerland) were maintained in a 1:1 mixture of DMEM and Ham's F12 complemented by 10% FBS, 1% non-essential amino acids and antibiotics. Both cell lines were tested for the absence of *Mycoplasma* infection and cultured to 90% confluence at 37°C in xenoestrogen-free plastic (Corning Inc., Grand Island, USA) under humidified air containing 5% CO_2.

Before each exposure to the chemicals, the growth medium was replaced by phenol red-free DMEM/F12 and cells were cultured for 48 h in the presence of 5% charcoal/dextran-stripped FBS (lacking estrogens or other growth factors that trigger the cell cycle), followed by the addition of acrylamide or glycidamide at the indicated concentrations. Glycidamide has been shown to be stable under these conditions (Silvari et al. 2005).

3.3. Cytotoxicity and caspase assays

A commercial kit was used to measure intracellular ATP levels. Briefly, MCF7 cells were grown in multi-well plates and exposed to the indicated concentrations of acrylamide or glycidamide. After 24 h, the CellTiter-Glo reagent (Promega) was added and the luminescent signal was recorded in a microplate reader following the manufacturer's instruction. The CellTiter 96 and CytoTox 96 assays (Promega) were used to monitor the metabolic activity and the release of lactate dehydrogenase. The luminescent Caspase-Glo assay (Promega) was used to determine the activity of caspases 3 and 7.

3.4. Gene expression analysis

After 24-h incubations with acrylamide or glycidamide, the cells were collected by trypsinization and total RNA was extracted with the RNeasy mini kit (Qiagen). The quality of RNA was determined on the Agilent Lab-on-a-chip Bioanalyzer 2000. Samples with a total area under the 28S and 18S bands of less than 65% of total RNA, as well as a 28S/18S ratio of less than 1.5, were considered to be degraded and therefore excluded from microarray analyses. The GeneChip Expression and IVT Labelling kits (Affymetrix) were used for the synthesis of complementary DNA and complementary RNA, respectively. The biotin-labeled RNA was fragmented and hybridized on Human Genome U122 plus 2.0 microarrays (Affymetrix) following the manufacturer's instructions.

After hybridization (16 h), the microarrays were processed by automated washing on the Affymetrix Fluidics Station 400. Staining of the hybridized probes was performed with fluorescent streptavidin-phycoerythrin conjugates (1 mg/ml; Molecular Probes). The subsequent scanning of DNA microarrays was carried out on an Affymetrix laser instrument. The data sets were normalized and analyzed using the GeneSpring 7.2

software (Silicon Genetics). The gene ontology database (www.geneontology.org) was consulted for the molecular function of each transcript.

3.5. Real-time quantitative RT-PCR

TaqMan gene expression assays containing pre-designed primers and probes for the selected transcripts and TaqMan universal PCR master mix were obtained from Applied Biosystems. Briefly, 100 ng of complementary DNA were mixed with 100 nM of forward and reverse primers in a final volume of 25 µl. The reactions were performed in an ABI PRISM 7700 Sequence Detection System (Applied Biosystems) in 45 cycles (95°C for 15 sec, 60°C for 1 min) after an initial 10-min incubation at 95°C. The fold change in the expression of each gene was calculated using the $2^{-\Delta\Delta C_T}$ method (Livak and Schmittgen 2001), with the glyceraldehyde-3-phosphate dehydrogenase (GAPDH) transcript as an endogenous control.

3.6. Glutathione assay

MCF7 or CaCo-2 cells were grown in 6-well plates until a confluence of 90%. After treatment with the indicated glycidamide concentrations (in 3 ml medium), 5×10^5 cells were washed with phosphate-buffered saline, deproteinated with 10 mM HCl, and lysed by freezing and thawing. The pH was neutralized with 5% (w/v) 5-sulfosalicylic acid dihydrate (Fluka). After centrifugation, reduced GSH in the supernatant was measured with the colorimetric QuantiChrom Glutathione Assay kit (BioAssay Systems, Hayward, USA) following the manufacturer's instructions.

3.7. NF-κB reporter assay

MCF7 cells (70% confluent) were co-transfected (jetPEI reagent, PolyPlus-Transfection, Illkirch, France) with the reporter construct pBII-Luc, carrying the firefly luciferase gene under control of NF-κB binding sites (Hassa et al. 2001), and the vector pRL-TK (Promega), which drives the constitutive expression of the *Renilla* luciferase. A pBII-Luc derivative lacking NF-κB binding sites was used to test the assay specificity. After transfection, cells were allowed to recover for 2 h before exposure to the indicated concentrations of glycidamide. Following varying incubation times, firefly and *Renilla* luciferase expression were determined in cell lysates using the Dual Luciferase system (Promega). Induction of the reporter gene was then calculated from the ratio of activity of the two enzymes.

4. RESULTS

4.1. Glycidamide toxicity

The dose range to be tested in the DNA microarray experiments has been determined using standard viability assays. Human MCF7 mammary tumor cells were exposed for 24 h to increasing concentrations of glycidamide or the parent compound acrylamide. Cell viability was tested by measuring the intracellular ATP concentration, which is used as an indicator of overall metabolic activity. The resulting dose response demonstrated that neither glycidamide nor acrylamide exerted cytotoxic effects at concentrations of up to 1 mM (Fig. 3). A significant reduction of ATP levels was observed only following the 10-mM glycidamide treatment.

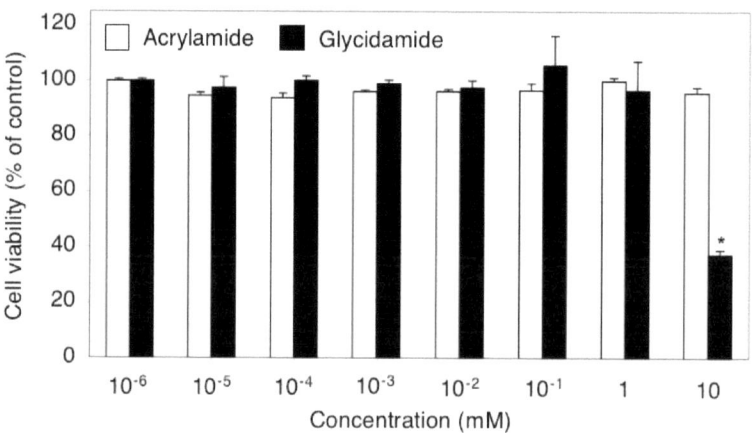

Figure 3. Cytotoxicity of acrylamide and glycidamide. Confluent MCF7 cell cultures were treated with increasing concentrations of each chemical for 24 h. Subsequently,

their metabolic activity was determined by measuring intracellular ATP pools and the results are expressed as the percentage of the ATP concentration found in untreated controls (mean of five independent determinations). Error bars = 95% confidence intervals. The asterisk indicates a statistically significant difference between cells treated with acrylamide or glycidamide at a 1-mM concentration (P < 0.05, Mann-Whitney U test).

Comparable results, i.e., no cytotoxicity at concentrations of up to 1 mM, were obtained when the metabolic activity was assessed with the tetrazolium reagent (MTT assay) or when cell lysis was measured by the release of lactate dehydrogenase into the cell culture supernatant (data not shown). In the same concentration range of up to 1 mM, there was no activation of caspases 3 and 7 following 24-h exposures to glycidamide and acrylamide (data not shown), suggesting that both compounds fail to induce an apoptotic response. These toxicity assays performed over short 24-h periods cannot exclude that cell survival may be affected after longer incubation times.

4.2. *Expression profiling*

High-density oligonucleotide microarray experiments were performed to determine global changes of gene expression in MCF7 cells. Each transcriptome was assessed in three independent experiments using separate cell cultures and RNA preparations. Following 24-h glycidamide or acrylamide treatments, the messenger RNA was analyzed on Affymetrix U122 plus 2.0 microarrays covering the sequences of ~47,000 human transcripts. Approximately 35% of all examined gene products were called to be present by the GeneChip Operating 3.0 software.

Fig. 4A compares the profiles of two independent experiments conducted with untreated MCF7 cells, i.e., in the absence of glycidamide or acrylamide stimulation. In this case, the data points accumulate along the diagonal axis of the scatter plot, thus illustrating that repeated microarray determinations yielded nearly identical results. These baseline values were then plotted against the transcriptional profiles obtained by exposing MCF7 cells to 1-mM concentrations of the test compounds. In the comparison between a representative control sample and the 1-mM glycidamide treatment, the cloud of data became much wider indicating that a large number of genes are either over- or underexpressed upon glycidamide exposure (Fig. 4B). In response to acrylamide, however, the expression values were closer to the baseline control (Fig. 4C), indicating that the parent compound itself induces less prominent changes of gene expression. In view of the more conspicuous transcriptional effects elicited by glycidamide, only the genomic response to this oxidative metabolite was further investigated at lower doses.

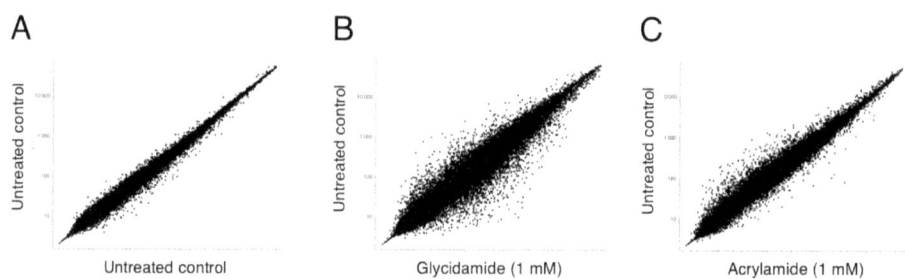

Figure 4. Overall expression changes. Each scatter plot shows the normalized data from individual hybridizations on Affymetrix high-density DNA microarrays. The messenger RNA levels are expressed in arbitrary units. *(A)* Comparison between the transcriptome of two independent samples of untreated MCF7 cells. *(B)* Comparison between an untreated control and MCF7 cells exposed to 1 mM glycidamide. *(C)* Comparison between the same untreated control and MCF7 cells treated with 1 mM acrylamide.

4.3. Multivariate analysis of transcriptomes

The GeneSpring 7.2 software was employed to integrate the hybridization intensities of triplicate experiments and to perform data analysis. The principal component analysis (PCA) constitutes a linear dimensionality reduction technique that is commonly applied to classify complex transcriptional patterns (Van der Werf et al. 2006). The resulting output can be visualized in two-dimensional plots, where each point represents the entire transcriptome of a single sample. Transcriptomes that cluster together are overall very similar, whereas transcriptional patterns that differ from each other are located further apart.

Fig. 5 demonstrates that all expression profiles obtained by exposing MCF7 cells to glycidamide, at concentrations between 1 µM and 1 mM, are clearly separated from the untreated controls, implying that the changes due to technical variation are less important than the gene regulation occurring in response to different concentrations of the test compound. Individual experiments from each treatment group cluster closely together but, with increasing glycidamide concentrations, we observed a gradual shift along the X-axis, which represents the component that accounts for the highest proportion (81.1%) of the total variance.

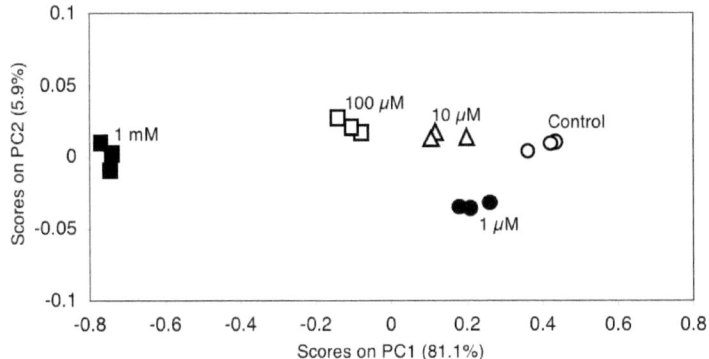

Figure 5. PCA plot of the transcription profiles in MCF7 cells exposed to increasing concentrations of glycidamide. Each treatment group consists of three independent experiments.

This principal component shows that the gene expression program of MCF7 cells is altered by glycidamide exposure in a dose-dependent manner. Interestingly, a minor component (PC2 on the Y-axis) accounts for only 5.9% of the total variance, although it clearly separates the 1-µM treatments from all other experiments.

4.4. Univariate transcriptome analysis

The fold differences for each detectable transcript were determined from the comparison between glycidamide-treated MCF7 cells and the reference values from unexposed controls. These differential expression data were filtered using, as thresholds, a fold change of > 3.0 and a statistical significance of $P < 0.05$ (two-sided ANOVA) in at least one of the treatment groups. The false discovery rate according to Benjamini and Hochberg (Benjamini and Hochberg, 1995) was < 0.1. This analysis yielded > 100 glycidamide-regulated transcripts that encode protein products whose known or inferred biological functions fall into three categories.

A major functional cluster comprises detoxification processes involving two routes of glycidamide inactivation, i.e., GSH conjugation and opening of the epoxide ring by epoxide hydrolases (Table 1A). In particular, the GSH system was modulated by overexpression of GCLM, a regulatory subunit that stimulates the cysteine ligase in catalyzing the rate-limiting step of GSH biosynthesis (Lee et al. 2006). The capacity of this pathway was further enhanced by the up-regulation of a membrane carrier (SLC7A11) that mediates the cellular uptake of cystine moieties required for GSH production (Huang et al. 2005).

Table 1A. *Regulation of transcripts coding for factors involved in detoxification (fold changes of expression relative to untreated controls). All concentrations tested in triplicates.*

Name	Description	Glycidamide (mM)			
		0.001	0.01	0.1	1
SLC7A11	Solute carrier family 7, member A11	1.4	1.5	1.6	37.3
AKR1B10	Aldo-keto reductase family 1, member B10	-2.4	-1.5	1.8	32.4
GPX2	Glutathione peroxidase 2	1.0	1.1	2.4	20.0
LTB4DH	Leukotriene B4 12-hydroxydehydrogenase	-1.4	-2.0	1.3	14.5
CYP4F11	Cytochrome P450, family 4, subfamily F, polypeptide 11	1.0	1.1	1.2	13.5
AKR1C3	Aldo-keto reductase family 1, member C3	1.2	1.1	1.2	10.6
ME1	Malic enzyme 1	-1.3	-1.5	1.9	7.8
AKR1C1	Aldo-keto reductase family 1, member C1	-1.5	-1.4	4.1	7.5
DHRS2	Dehydrogenase/reductase (SDR family) member 2	1.1	1.0	1.0	7.5
AKR1C2	Aldo-keto reductase family 1, member C2	-1.2	1.2	1.8	6.2
GCLM	Glutamate-cysteine ligase, modifier subunit	-1.3	-1.3	1.4	6.2
GPX3	Glutathione peroxidase 3	1.5	-1.2	1.0	6.0
EPHX1	Epoxide hydrolase 1	1.2	1.8	1.2	5.2
MGST1	Microsomal glutathione S-transferase 1	1.2	1.2	1.3	4.9
CBR1	Carbonyl reductase 1	1.5	1.0	1.6	4.4
CBR3	Carbonyl reductase 3	1.3	-1.1	1.0	4.2
G6PD	Glucose-6-phosphate dehydrogenase	1.2	1.4	1.0	4.2
SULT1A3,4	Sulfotransferase family 1A, member 3 and 4	1.7	1.2	1.1	3.4
ESD	Esterase D/formylglutathione hydrolase	1.4	1.1	1.4	3.2
SULT1A1	Sulfotransferase family 1A, member 1	1.7	1.1	1.1	3.1
CYP4B1	Cytochrome P450, family 4, subfamily B, polypeptide 1	1.1	-1.5	-1.6	-19.0
CYP1B1	Cytochrome P450, family 1, subfamily B, polypeptide 1	-2.0	-1.7	-1.4	-18.5
ALDH3B2	Aldehyde dehydrogenase 3 family, member B2	-1.2	-1.1	-1.4	-15.5
ALDH4A1	Aldehyde dehydrogenase 4 family, member A1	-1.2	-1.3	-1.5	-4.6
CYP1A1	Cytochrome P450, family 1, subfamily A, polypeptide 1	-1.7	-4.5	-7.0	-4.0
IDH2	Isocitrate dehydrogenase, mitochondrial	1.2	-1.1	-1.2	-3.5
CYP2J2	Cytochrome P450, family 2, subfamily J, polypeptide 2	1.6	1.1	-1.1	-3.2

As shown in Table 1A, glycidamide exposure led to transcriptional induction of the following other members of the GSH system: a transferase that catalyzes the conjugation of toxicants to the GSH moiety (MGST1), two distinct GSH peroxidases (GPX2 and GPX3), and metabolic enzymes (ME1, G6PD) that contribute to NADPH synthesis, thereby promoting the turnover of oxidized GSSG. Further effects of glycidamide treatment include the overexpression of reductases (DHRS2, AKR1B10, AKR1C1, AKR1C2, AKR1C3, LTB4DH, CBR1, CBR3 and ESD) that protect the organism from toxic carbonyl compounds (Dick et al. 2001; Covarrubias et al. 2006). Finally, we observed that one representative of the cytochrome P450 superfamily (CYP4F11) was overexpressed, whereas CYP1A1, CYP1B1, CYP2J2 and CYP4B1 were transcriptionally repressed in glycidamide-treated cells. A comparison with the 1-mM acrylamide treatment (Fig. 4C) showed that many of these glycidamide-responsive transcripts were also regulated by acrylamide, but with amplitudes of induction or repression that were at least four times lower than those observed with an equivalent concentration of glycidamide (data not shown).

The second functional cluster involves a dual response to oxidative stress (Table 1B). One part of this reaction is the induction of intracellular antioxidants such as the thioredoxin/thioredoxin reductase system, sulfiredoxin (SRXN1) and peroxiredoxins (PRDX3 and PRDX6). Lipoic acid synthase (LIAS) contributes to the same cytoprotective mechanism as this enzyme catalyzes the synthesis of lipoic acid, a potent natural antioxidant (Yi and Maeda 2005). In addition, cells react to oxidative stress by removing damaged protein aggregates. This response is evidenced by the induction of a ubiquitin-dependent protease (USP40) as well as by the overexpression of components of the autophagic system (APG3, CLTC and SQSTM1). Another transcript overexpressed in glycidamide-treated cells codes for MAFG, which is one of the MAF proteins that are essential for the induction of antioxidant factors (Katsuoka et al. 2005). Finally, we observed that glycidamide treatment stimulates the expression of EME1, a key DNA repair endonuclease (McPherson et al. 2004).

Table 1B. *Regulation of factors involved in the oxidative stress response (fold changes of expression relative to untreated controls). All concentrations tested in triplicates.*

Name	Description	Glycidamide (mM)			
		0.001	0.01	0.1	1
MTABC3	Mammalian mitochondrial ABP protein 3	1.1	1.0	1.4	16.5
USP40	Ubiquitin-specific protease 40	1.2	1.4	1.6	6.1
TXNRD1	Thioredoxin reductase 1	-2.9	-2.9	1.5	6.0
APG3	Autophagy Apg3p/Aut1p-like	-1.2	-1.2	1.1	6.0
HMOX	Heme oxygenase 1	1.0	1.0	1.2	5.7
CLTC	Clathrin, heavy polipeptide	1.5	1.0	1.4	5.1
SRXN1	Sulfiredoxin 1	-1.3	-1.5	1.3	5.0
NQO1	NAD(P)H dehydrogenase, quinone 1	-1.1	-1.5	1.7	4.5
FTH1	Ferritin, heavy polypeptide 1	-1.6	-1.1	1.2	4.1
PRDX6	Peroxiredoxin 6	1.2	-1.6	-1.3	3.9
MAFG	Sushi domain containing 4	-1.1	-1.3	1.1	3.8
EME1	Essential meiotic endonuclease 1	-1.2	2.1	2.8	3.7
TXN	Thioredoxin	1.7	1.4	2.0	3.6
LIAS	Lipoic acid synthetase	1.6	-1.2	1.2	3.6
SQSTM1	Sequestosome 1	-1.6	-1.3	1.2	3.4
FECH	Ferrochetalase	1.2	1.1	1.2	3.4
PRDX3	Peroxiredoxin 3	1.4	1.1	1.2	3.3
SELENBP1	Selenium binding protein 1	1.2	1.0	-1.3	-7.5
SEPP1	Selenoprotein P, plasma, 1	-1.1	-1.1	-1.4	-8.3

The third functional cluster is related to cancer progression (Table 1C). Glycidamide exposure of MCF7 cells resulted in the transcriptional regulation of many genes linked to malignancy or tissue invasion, including the growth factors OPG, ARC, HIP, KITLG, METAP2, and the insulin-like growth factor (IGF) receptor IGFR2 (see discussion). The response to glycidamide is further characterized by the down-regulation of transcripts coding for cell adhesion molecules, including ITGB6, CDH12, CTNND2, ITGA6, SHANK2 and ANKRD34 (Table 1C). This same endpoint is favored by the induction of TRPM7, which suppresses cell adhesion (Su et al. 2006), and the transcriptional down-regulation of tissue inhibitors of metalloproteinases (TIMP3, TIMP2). The growth-inhibitory factors ING3, CASP7 and GADD45B were underexpressed. In addition, a Medline search showed that many other down-regulated transcripts (SASH1, PGM2L1, PACE4, CAV1, PRLR, DOCK8, CA12, CRABP2, WWOX, PTPN13 and ST7; bottom of Table 1C) have previously been associated with the suppression of cell transformation and tumor progression.

Table 1C. *Regulation of transcripts linked to cancer progression (fold changes of expression relative to untreated controls). All concentrations tested in triplicates.*

Name	Description	Glycidamide (mM)			
		0.001	0.01	0.1	1
TD2L	Tumor differentially expressed 2 like	1.3	1.3	1.1	11.9
RANK	Receptor activator of NF-κB	1.7	-1.9	1.2	8.7
HNLF	Putative NF-κB activating protein HNLF	1.6	1.4	1.6	7.8
TRPM7	Transient receptor potential cation channel	1.6	2.1	1.6	5.2
OPG	Osteoprotegerin	-1.7	-1.6	1.1	5.2
COMMD10	COMM domain containing 10, a NF-κB inhibitor	1.0	-1.2	1.0	4.7
CAPN7	Calpain 7	1.1	2.0	1.5	4.1
HIP14	Huntingtin interacting protein 14	1.6	1.5	1.4	3.9
CCNI	Cyclin I	1.1	1.1	1.0	3.6
TNFSF9	Tumor necrosis factor (ligand) superfamily, member 9	1.0	-1.1	1.3	3.6
MAPK12	Mitogen-activated protein kinase 12	1.0	1.0	1.0	3.3
TNFRSF25	Tumor necrosis factor receptor superfamily, member 25	1.0	1.0	1.0	3.1
IGF2R	Insulin-like growth factor 2 receptor	1.3	1.3	1.4	3.1
METAP2	Methionyl aminopeptidase 2	1.3	1.2	1.1	3.1
ARC	Apoptosis repressor with caspase-resistant domain	1.7	1.1	1.3	3.0
KITLG	KIT ligand	-1.1	1.1	1.2	3.0
ITGB6	Integrin, beta 6	1.2	-1.8	-1.6	-63.6
ANXA1	Annexin A1	1.1	1.2	-1.6	-38.3

IL1R1	Interleukin 1 receptor type 1	-1.1	-1.8	-1.8	-24.3
WISP2	WNT1 inducible signalling pathway protein 2	1.1	-2.3	-1.9	-22.0
IGFBP4	Insulin-like growth factor binding protein 4	3.9	1.2	-2.0	-21.9
TM4SF1	Transmembrane superfamily member 1	-1.2	-1.4	-1.9	-18.4
HS6ST2	Heparan sulfate 6-O-sulfotransferase 2	-1.2	-1.8	-3.2	-18.1
IFITM1	Interferon-induced transmembrane protein 1	-1.1	-1.2	-2.4	-17.3
SASH1	SAM and SH3 domain containing 1	-1.7	-1.1	-1.1	-17.0
TIMP3	Tissue inhibitor of metalloproteinase 3	-1.5	1.2	-1.6	-14.6
IGFBP5	Insulin-like growth factor binding protein 5	1.5	-1.2	-1.4	-13.0
PGM2L1	Phosphoglucomutase 2-like 1	-1.6	-1.7	-1.1	-10.9
SIDT1	SID1 transmembrane family member 1	-1.1	-1.3	-1.4	-10.7
PACE4	Paired basic amino acid cleaving system 4	-1.4	-1.5	-1.1	-10.1
CAV1	Caveolin 1	1.7	-1.6	-1.4	-9.5
CDH12	Cadherin 12, type 2 (N-cadherin 2)	-1.1	-1.0	-1.1	-8.1
PRLR	Prolactin receptor	1.3	-1.1	-1.4	-7.7
SELENBP1	Selenium binding protein 1	1.2	1.0	-1.3	-7.5
DOCK8	Dedicator of cytokinesis 8	-1.1	-1.7	-1.1	-7.4
CAPN2	Calpain 2 lage subunit	-1.3	-3.7	-3.7	-6.6
SIAT4A	Sialyltransferase 4A	1.7	1.9	1.2	6.4
FHOD3	Formin homology 2 domain containing 3	-1.2	-6.2	-4.9	-6.2
CA12	Carboanhydrase XII	1.0	-1.5	-1.1	-6.0
CRABP2	Cellular retinoic acid binding protein 2	1.3	1.3	-1.4	-6.0
ING3	Inhibitor of growth family, member 3	-1.1	-1.4	1.2	-5.9
CTNND2	Catenin (Cadherin associated protein), delta 2	-1.5	-2.0	-1.2	-5.5
CAV2	Caveolin 2	1.2	-1.6	-1.4	-5.5
WWOX	WW domain containing oxidoreductase	1.1	1.0	1.0	-5.3
PTPN13	Protein tyrosine phosphatase, non-receptor type 13	1.0	-1.4	-1.2	-5.0
SHANK2	SH3 and multiple ankyrin repeat domains 2	-1.4	-1.6	-1.1	-4.6
CAPN13	Calpain 13	1.0	1.0	-1.3	-4.0
TMEM46	Transmembrane protein 46	-1.2	-1.6	-1.9	-4.0
TMPRSS2	Transmembrane protease serine 2	-1.1	-1.7	-1.3	-4.0
IGFBP2	Insulin-like growth factor binding protein 2	1.7	-1.2	-1.6	-3.9
ITGA6	Integrin, alpha 6	-1.3	-3.4	-4.0	-3.8
CASP7	Caspase 7, apoptosis-related cysteine protease	-1.1	-1.2	-1.1	-3.8
TIMP2	Tissue inhibitor of metalloproteinase 2	-1.2	-3.9	-2.5	-3.8
ANKRD34	Ankyrin repeat domain 34	1.3	1.1	1.1	-3.7
ST7	Suppression of tumorigenicity 7	-1.7	-2.3	-2.4	-3.4

TRAF5	TNF receptor-associated factor 5	-1.1	-1.2	1.0	-3.4
GADD45B	Growth arrest and DNA-damage-inducible, beta	1.3	-1.1	-1.2	-3.3
MMP16	Matrix metalloproteinase 16 (membrane-inserted)	1.2	1.3	-1.1	-3.1

4.5. Data verification by RT-PCR analysis

DNA microarry hybridization is a multiple-comparison procedure with an inherent false discovery rate (Benjamini and Hochberg 1995). Therefore, it is necessary to validate the microarray results with a quantitative method targeted to single endpoints. First, real-time reverse transcriptase (RT)-PCR determinations were carried out on 16 transcripts using the RNA samples obtained from the previous high-dose experiments with 100 µM and 1 mM glycidamide. After normalization with the GAPDH (glyceraldehyde-3-phosphate dehydrogenase) housekeeping control, expression values were determined as the ratio of messenger level between glycidamide-exposed and untreated cells. A direct comparison of the microarray hybridization results with the respective RT-PCR values revealed a high degree of correlation for the transcripts that were regulated by the glycidamide stimulus in a significant manner. The only exception among the 16 tested mRNAs was the BRCA2 transcript, for which a more moderate induction was found by RT-PCR than in the microarray hybridizations (data not shown).

The same transcripts (except the BRCA2 messenger) were further analyzed to verify the reproducibility of these findings. For that purpose, the treatment of MCF7 cells was repeated with a new series of triplicate experiments, thus generating an independent set of samples for RT-PCR analysis. After normalization against the GAPDH housekeeping control, the expression values were again transformed to ratios between glycidamide-exposed and untreated cells. The results of Fig. 4A show that, as it was found by microarray hybridizations, some transcripts were consistently up-regulated following a treatment with only 1 µM glycidamide. Examples of this low-dose response are EPHX1 (an epoxide hydrolase) and SLC7A11. Additional experiments conducted with even lower toxicant levels showed that EPHX1 is significantly ($P < 0.001$) up-regulated by a factor of 1.6 ± 0.05 following a 0.1-μM glycidamide treatment. Other transcripts (EME1, GCLM or AKR1C2) were down-regulated in the presence of 1 μM glycidamide, but up-regulated at higher concentrations (see Tables 1A-C and Fig. 4A). On the other hand, the FHOD3 transcript (coding for a putative regulator of actin function; Katoh and Katoh 2004) was down-regulated at all glycidamide concentrations of 1 μM or higher (Table 2A).

Table 2A. Quantification of the MCF7 microarray data by real-time RT-PCR. Analysis of 15 representative transcripts 10 of which were found to be up-regulated after a 1-mM glycidamide exposure and 5 of which were found to be down-regulated by the 1-mM exposure to glycidamide in the previous microarray determinations. All results (fold changes relative to untreated controls) are shown as the mean values of three independent determinations. The standard deviations of the three fold change values are indicated in brackets. Asterisks indicate values that are significantly different from the unexposed controls ($P < 0.05$, Mann-Whitney U test).

Name	Description	Glycidamide (mM)			
		0.001	0.01	0.1	1
		(Stdev)	(Stdev)	(Stdev)	(Stdev)
GPX2	Gutathione peroxidase 2	-1.02	1.11*	2.37*	81.19*
		(0.004)	(0.035)	(0.176)	(3.268)
SLC7A11	Solute carrier family 7, member A11	1.43*	1.54*	2.14*	41.84*
		(0.123)	(0.035)	(0.060)	(1.174)
AKR1C3	Aldo-keto reductase family 1, member C3	1.19	1.12*	1.93*	20.4*
		(0.095)	(0.047)	(0.281)	(1.555)
AKR1C2	Aldo-keto reductase family 1, member C2	-1.25	1.23*	1.6	19.95*
		(0.328)	(0.064)	(0.346)	(3.447)
EPHX1	Epoxide hydrolase 1	1.55*	1.5*	1.37	9.69*
		(0.040)	(0.055)	(0.105)	(1.845)
GCLM	Glutamate-cysteine ligase, modifier subunit	-1.28	-1.29	1.18	8.55*

			(0.031)	(0.118)	(0.125)	(1.158)
CYP4F11	Cytochrom P450, family 4, subfamily F, polypeptide 11	1.03	1.12	1	7.36*
		(0.191)	(0.078)	(0.070)	(0.144)
RRM2	Ribonucleotide reductase M2 polypeptide	1.35	1.15*	1*	2.83*
		(0.166)	(0.012)	(0.354)	(0.359)
TXN	Thioredoxin	1.07	1	1.11	2.3*
		(0.037)	(0.002)	(0.056)	(0.171)
EME1	Endomeiotic endonuclease 1	-1.17*	-1.01	1.24*	2.27*
		(0.042)	(0.122)	(0.067)	(0.229)
FHOD3	Formin homology domain containing 3	-1.30*	-1.30	-1.89*	-66.67*
		(0.044)	(0.159)	(0.131)	(0.003)
ITGB6	Integrin beta 6	1.17	1.42	-1.79*	-35.71*
		(0.036)	(0.163)	(0.035)	(0.002)
CAPN13	Calpain 13	1	1	-1.30*	-30.30*
		(0.032)	(0.046)	(0.060)	(0.004)
CDH12	Cadherin 12	-1.14*	1.20	-1.15	-12.94*
		(0.046)	(0.136)	(0.115)	(0.0003)
ANXA1	Annexin A1	1.06	1.16	-2.27*	-12.82*
		(0.059)	(0.140)	(0.021)	(0.015)

We next extended this RT-PCR analysis to the human colonic cell line CaCo-2, which has been shown to mimic the absorptive properties of a differentiated intestinal epithelium (Meunier et al. 1995). Interestingly, we found that CaCo-2 cells react to glycidamide with a transcriptional response that largely overlaps with that observed in MCF7 cells. Examples of this convergent regulation in the two different cell lines include the overexpression of SLC7A11, GCLM, CYP4F11, AKR1C3, and GPX2, and the common underexpression of ITGB6 and CAPN13 (Table 2B). ANXA1 was down-regulated in MCF7 but up-regulated in CaCo-2 cells. Some other transcripts (AKR1C2, CDH12 and FHOD3) turned out to be absent in CaCo-2 cells.

Table 2B. *Quantification by real-time RT-PCR (CaCo2). The 15 transcripts verified in MCF7 by Real-time PCR were tested in the CaCo2 cell line. 6 of them were found to be up-regulated after a 1-mM glycidamide exposure and 2 of them were found to be down-regulated by the 1-mM exposure to glycidamide. All results (fold changes relative to untreated controls) are shown as the mean values of three independent determinations. The standard deviations of the three fold change values are indicated in brackets. . Asterisks indicate values that are significantly different from the unexposed controls (P < 0.05, Mann-Whitney U test).*

Name	Description	Glycidamide (mM)			
		0.001	0.01	0.1	1
		(Stdev)	(Stdev)	(Stdev)	(Stdev)
SLC7A11	Solute carrier family 7, member A11	-1.20	-1.03	1.78*	15.24*
		(0.052)	(0.024)	(0.087)	(0.597)
GCLM	Glutamate-cysteine ligase, modifier subunit	-1.54*	-1.57	-1.11	10.56*
		(0.012)	(0.004)	(0.927)	(0.001)
CYP4F11	Cytochrom P450, family 4, subfamily F, polypeptide 11	1.00	1.11*	-4.85*	7.38*
		(0.108)	(0.035)	(0.065)	(1.726)
AKR1C3	Aldo-keto reductase family 1, member C3	1.04	1.05	1.573*	7.26*
		(0.104)	(0.032)	(0.011)	(0.313)
ANXA1	Annexin A1	-1.96*	-1.79*	-1.63*	3.97*
		(0.035)	(0.063)	(0.024)	(0.176)
GPX2	Glutathione peroxidase 2	-1.45*	-1.01	1.44*	3.46*
		(0.057)	(0.131)	(0.088)	(0.176)
ITGB6	Integrin beta 6	-1.10*	-1.30*	-1.23*	-5.05*
		(0.023)	(0.073)	(0.025)	(0.021)
CAPN13	Calpain 13	1.00	1.10	1.01	-3.56*
		(0.046)	(0.075)	(0.018)	(0.023)

4.6. Changes of GSH status

Considering that many factors involved in the GSH system are induced upon glycidamide treatment (Table 1A), we tested the consequence of glycidamide exposure on the effective intracellular GSH level. Approximately 3 million cells (corresponding to a total intracellular volume of about 3 µl) were exposed to medium (3 ml) containing increasing concentrations of glycidamide or acrylamide. Interestingly, we found that the GSH pool of MCF7 cells was partially depleted after a 24-h incubation with 1 µM glycidamide (Fig. 6A). At higher concentrations, the normal GSH concentration was gradually reconstituted and, after a 1-mM glycidamide exposure, the GSH pool of MCF7 cells reached a higher level than in the untreated controls.

Similarly, CaCo-2 cells respond to 1-µM and 10-µM treatments with a significant depression of GSH pools. Again, normal GSH levels were restored with increasing glycidamide concentrations (Fig. 6B). These results indicate that the transcriptional induction of key factors responsible for GSH biosynthesis and recycling compensates for the partial GSH loss due to S-conjugation with the toxic metabolite. Consistent with its more limited transcriptional effects (Fig. 4C), no reparation of the GSH pool was observed upon acrylamide treatment of MCF7 (Fig. 6C) or CaCo-2 cells (Fig. 6D).

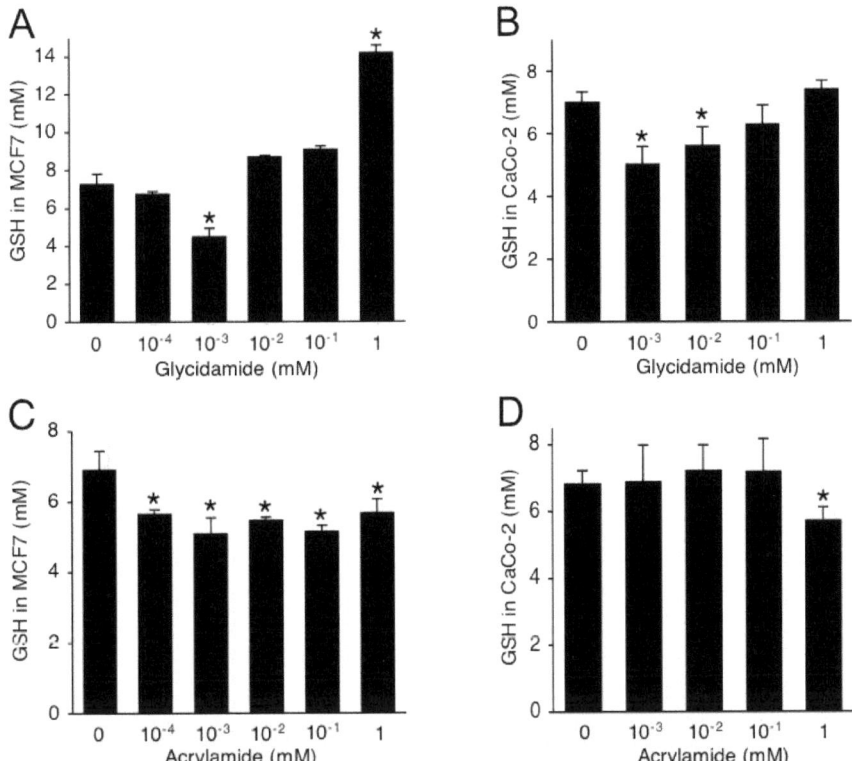

Figure 6. Measurement of GSH pools and NF-κB activity. (**A**) GSH levels in MCF7 cells after 24-h exposures to the indicated glycidamide concentrations. (**B**) GSH levels in CaCo-2 cells following glycidamide treatments. (**C**) GSH levels in MCF7 cells after 24-h exposures to the indicated acrylamide concentrations. (**D**) GSH levels in CaCo-2 cells following acrylamide treatments. All GSH quantifications are shown as the mean of five independent measurements. Error bars indicate the standard deviation, asterisks indicate values that are significantly different from the unexposed controls ($P < 0.05$, Mann-Whitney U test).

4.7. NF-κB activation

Glycidamide exposure results in the stimulation of both positive and negative regulators of the NF-κB pathway. In fact, the up-regulation of transcripts coding for RANK and HNLF, which activate NF-κB, is accompanied by the concomitant overexpression of inhibitors of the NF-κB pathway such as OPG or COMMD10 (Table 1C). In view of these opposite effects, we performed a functional assay, based on an exogenous reporter gene, to determine how the NF-κB status is altered after glycidamide exposure. For that purpose, MCF7 cells were transiently transfected with a construct that carries the DNA sequence for firefly luciferase under the control of a minimal promoter containing wild-type NF-κB binding sites (Hassa et al. 2001). This reporter gene assay yielded a dose-dependent activation of NF-κB in response to glycidamide, with a substantial effect already detectable after the 1-μM treatment (Fig. 7A). In time course experiments, NF-κB activity peaked after 12 h of glycidamide exposure (Fig. 7B). No reporter gene induction was detected in the presence of a control vector where the NF-κB binding sites had been omitted (data not shown). In summary, this functional assay revealed that the stress-induced activation of NF-κB prevails over its negative regulators, thus resulting in an increased constitutive activity of this key transcription factor.

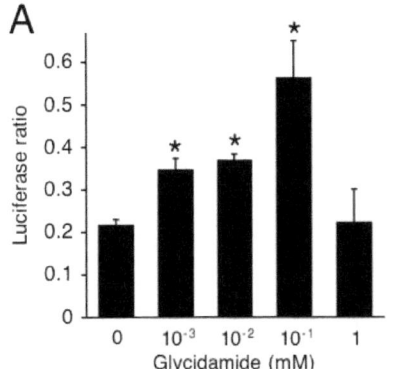 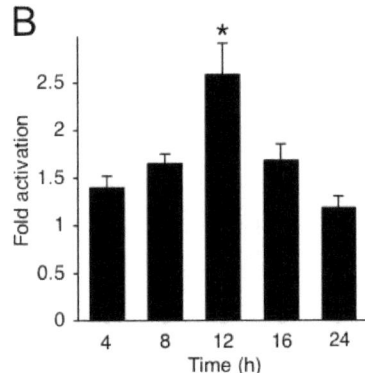

Figure 7. *(A) Reporter gene assay demonstrating NF-κB activation after 12-h treatments with glycidamide. The results are shown as the ratio between the reporter gene (firefly luciferase) activity and the internal Renilla standard (five independent determinations). (B) Time course of NF-κB activation in MCF7 cells treated with 100 μM glycidamide (3 independent experiments). Error bars = 95% confidence intervals. Asterisks indicate values that are significantly different from the unexposed controls ($P < 0.05$, Mann-Whitney U test).*

5. DISCUSSION

Genome-wide transcriptomes have been determined with high-density DNA microarrays to monitor the dose-dependent response of human cells to glycidamide, the reactive oxidative metabolite generated from acrylamide. It is expected that glycidamide concentrations of 10 µM or higher exceed the estimated dose levels that may occur in humans. Recent studies have shown that oral administration of a single 0.1 mg/kg acrylamide bolus to rodents resulted in blood and tissue peak concentrations of up to 1 µM glycidamide (Doerge et al. 2005). Here, our quantitative RT-PCR assays demonstrated that changes of gene expression with up to 2-fold inductions or repressions could be observed following a 1-µM glycidamide treatment, thus approaching the concentration range that is relevant for the assessment of human health risks. Examples include the induction of transcripts coding for EPHX1 and SLC7A11, involved in detoxification processes, or the repression of CDH12 and FHOD3, implicated in tumor cell mobility and tissue invasion (Katoh and Katoh 2004). These RT-PCR determinations showed that many of the same transcriptional changes also occur in CaCo-2 cells, which are used as a surrogate for the human intestinal epithelium.

The micromolar doses of glycidamide that induce most of these transcriptional responses might still seem too high to be achieved by dietary exposure. However, the sensitivity of target cells depends on the capacity of their detoxification systems and, considering that the uptake of acrylamide is normally accompanied by other toxic food constituents that may saturate the cytoprotective systems, adverse effects are likely to occur at even lower concentrations than those expected from threshold experiments performed with a single compound. In the case of EPHX1, a significant transcriptional induction was observed at a glycidamide level of as low as 0.1 µM, indicating that this primary detoxification enzyme represents a sensitive biomarker for glycidamide exposure.

The principal advantage of obtaining a broad molecular fingerprint involving multiple simultaneous endpoints, as opposed to the determination of a single endpoint, is that the cellular response becomes more specific and sensitive. In fact, by screening for sets of transcripts that are up- or down-regulated in a coordinated manner, the global expression analysis has been shown to generate characteristic molecular signatures that improve the overall signal-to-noise ratio, thereby facilitating the assessment of biological effects. Even if at the single gene level there are only subtle differences in expression, the concordant regulation of multiple transcripts contributing to the same pathway may significantly alter cellular functions and, as a consequence, elicit a relevant response (Subramanian et al. 2005). By focusing on groups of genes that participate in common pathways, the detection of transcriptional patterns in target tissues generates a molecular signature that may replace more traditional biomarkers that rely on the measurement of macromolecular lesions or metabolic by-products with uncertain significance.

Our large-scale transcriptional analysis revealed that three major systems are regulated upon glycidamide treatment: detoxification (Table 1A), antioxidant defense (Table 1B) and tumor progression (Table 1C). One outstanding response to the oxidative imbalance generated by glycidamide is the overexpression of multiple members of the GSH pathway.

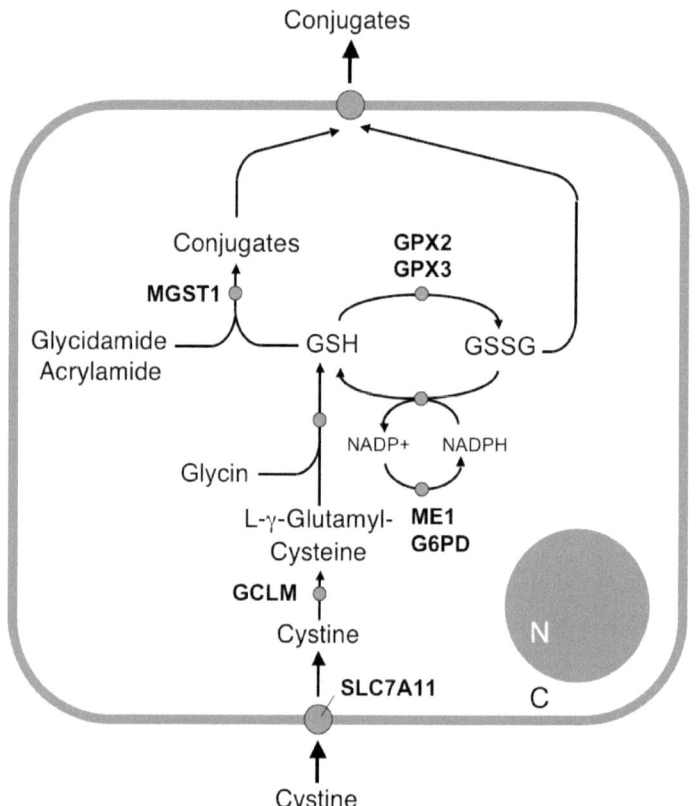

Figure 8. Scheme illustrating the different members of the GSH system leading to acrylamide and glycidamide detoxification that are subjected to transcriptional regulation following glycidamide treatment inside a mammalian cell. MGST = microsomal glutathione S-transferase; GPX = glutathione peroxidase; ME1 = malic enzyme 1; G6PD = glucose-6-phosphate dehydrogenase; GCLM = glutamate-cysteine ligase, modifier subunit; SLC7A11 = solute carrier family 7, member A11; N = nucleus, C = cytoplasm.

As illustrated in Fig. 8, these factors mediate not only GSH biosynthesis (SLC7A11, GCLM), but also subsequent conjugation (MGST1, GPX2, GPX3) and recycling steps (ME1, G6PD). Direct measurements in both MCF7 and CaCo-2 cells yielded a partial GSH depletion after a 24-h incubation with glycidamide, but only at the lower 0.1- or 1-µM concentration levels. In conjunction with the low-dose EPHX1 induction, this effect on the cellular thiol pool suggests a concentration range in which glycidamide is effectively inactivated inside the tested human cells. This cytoprotective window coincides with the results of the PCA analysis (Fig. 3), which indicates that the transcriptome generated by a 1-µM glycidamide treatment displays, in part, a different pattern than the profiles induced at higher doses.

Additional expression changes are observed at glycidamide concentrations of 10 µM or higher. An intriguing response is the up-regulation of several aldo-keto reductases (AKR1C1, AKR1C2 and AKR1C3) that have been implicated in breast and prostate cancer by virtue of their ability to catalyze the conversion of inactive androgen and estrogen precursors to biologically potent steroid hormones such as testosterone, 3α- and 3β-androstanediol, and 17β-estradiol (Lin et al. 2004). A hormonal activity of acrylamide or glycidamide, which may enhance their genotoxic properties, has already been discussed in view of the rodent long-term studies yielding tumors in endocrine glands and hormone-dependent tissues, including testicular mesotheliomas as well as mammary adenomas and carcinomas (Rice 2005). However, no data was provided to support an endocrine mode of action for acrylamide or glycidamide. Thus, the present report presents the first example of a hormonal dysregulation, involving the up-regulation of aldo-keto reductases, that may link acrylamide exposure to the development of tumors in steroid-dependent tissues.

Many other transcripts positively regulated by glycidamide (at concentrations of 10 µM or higher) have been associated with cancer progression (see Table 1C). For example, osteoprotegerin (OPG) has been reported to represent a survival factor in breast cancer tissue by acting as a soluble decoy receptor that blocks apoptosis-inducing signals such as TRAIL (Van Poznac et al. 2006). An anti-apoptotic activity has also been attributed to ARC (Neuss et al. 2001). Huntingtin interacting protein 14 (HIP) is a palmitoyltransferase enzyme that induces anchorage-independent cell growth (Ducker et al. 2004). Cell proliferation may be further stimulated by overexpression of the insulin-like growth factor (IGF) receptor IGFR2 and the concomitant down-regulation of IGFBP2, IGFBP4 and IGFBP5, which are known to attenuate IGF activity. KITLG is another growth factor overexpressed in glycidamide-treated cells. METAP2, induced by glycidamide exposure, has been associated with the metastatic progression of adenocarcinomas (Selvakumar et al. 2004). The high-dose response to glycidamide is further characterized by the down-regulation of transcripts coding for cell adhesion molecules and many other growth-inhibitory factors (Table 1C).

We found that multiple glycidamide-inducible genes code for members of the NF-κB pathway, a key mediator of cellular stress responses. A subsequent reporter gene assay in MCF7 mammary cells demonstrated that glycidamide treatment increases the constitutive activity of the NF-κB complex. NF-κB is known to trigger anti-apoptotic responses thereby controlling the ability of tumors to escape apoptosis-based surveillance mechanisms. NF-κB has also been implicated in the regulation of cell proliferation, angiogenesis, tumor cell migration and invasiveness (Karin 2006). An immediate clinical implication of overactive NF-κB complexes is illustrated by the finding that the constitutive stimulation of NF-κB is linked to a subset of high-risk breast cancers with poor prognosis (Zhou et al. 2006).

To conclude, this functional genomic study revealed that glycidamide exerts a plethora of transcriptional effects that should be included in risk assessment studies. As a consequence, we propose to implement a threshold level that prevents the induction of potentially hazardous transcriptional responses mediated by glycidamide in target tissues such as the mammary gland or the intestinal epithelium. The results of this in vitro study suggest that low-dose responses, primarily the induction of EPHX1, may exert beneficial effects by promoting inactivation of the toxicant, and that potentially adverse changes, for example dysregulation of steroid hormone synthesis, are detected at concentrations above the range that is relevant for human populations.

6. SIGNIFICANCE

Substantial efforts have been made during the last few years to investigate the possible hazardous effect of acrylamide occurring in food. A major gap of knowledge was the lack of information regarding the non-genotoxic effects of acrylamide in human cells. Thus, our aim was to provide the transcriptomic fingerprint induced by acrylamide or its metabolite glycidamide to enlighten the mode of action of these compounds and the cellular reactions they elicit.

Our transcriptomic approach revealed that glycidamide, the oxidative metabolite of acrylamide, causes broad alterations of genome function, thereby inducing distinctive expression profiles that may modulate the genotoxic effects of this food contaminant. By inspection of the dose-dependent cellular reactions, we concluded that low-dose responses (primarily the induction of EPHX1) exert beneficial effects by promoting inactivation of the toxicant (Fig. 9). Other detoxification processes observed at the low-dose glycidamide level of 0.1 µM include its inactivation through conjugation with glutathione. Adverse effects, such as for example the down-regulation of cell-adhesion molecules (CDH12, ANXA1, ITGB6), the up-regulation of factors that lead to dysregulation of steroid hormone synthesis (AKR1C2, AKR1C3), or factors that promote cell survival and cell cycle progression (NF-κB, RRM2, Cyclin-1, MAPK12) are detected at concentrations above the range that appears to be relevant for human populations. An induction of the DNA repair enzyme EME1, indicative of the formation of DNA damage, is also observed in the upper level of the tested dose range. Thus, the main implication of these findings for risk assessment is that transcriptional signatures associated with DNA damage or tumor cell progression may be expected only at doses that exceed the range of ordinary dietary exposure.

These findings indicate that the standard procedure of extrapolating from high-dose effects in rodents or other experimental systems to the very low-dose level of human exposure would lead to an overestimation of the toxicological risk, thus exaggerating the health hazards resulting from the presence of acrylamide in food and its metabolic conversion to glycidamide in the human body.

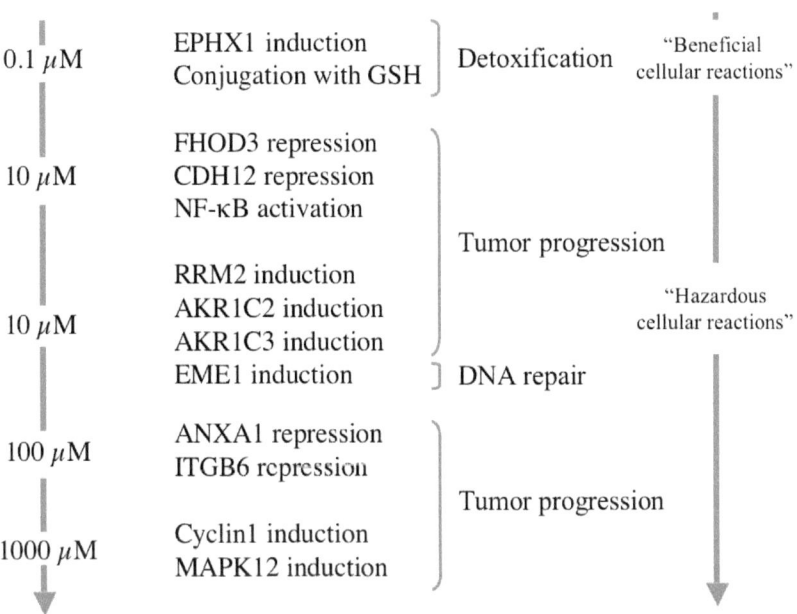

Figure 9. Summary of the main findings from the transcriptomic profiling of glycidamide effects in human cells. Beneficial responses are observed at the low-dose level, potentially hazardous effects are detected at high glycidamide concentrations. Abbreviations: EPHX1, epoxide hydrolase-1; GSH, glutathione; FHOD3, formin homology-3; CDH12, cadherin-12; NF-κB, nuclear factor-κB; RRM2, ribonucleotide reductase polypeptide-M2; AKR1C2, aldo-keto reductase-C2; AKR1C3, aldo-keto reductase-C3; EME1, essential meiotic endonuclease-1; ANXA1, annexin-A1; ITGB6, integrin beta-6; MAPK12, mitogen-activated protein kinase-12.

7. REFERENCES

Baum, M., Fauth, E., Fritzen, S. et al. (2005). Acrylamide and glycidamide: genotoxic effects in V79-cells and human blood. Mutation Research 580:61-69.

Benjamini, Y., Hochberg, Y. (1995). Controlling the false discovery rate: a practical and powerful approach to multiple testing. Journal of the Royal Statistical Society 57:289-300.

Bergmark, E. (1997). Hemoglobin adducts of acrylamide and acrylonitrile in laboratory workers, smokers and nonsmokers. Chemical Research in Toxicology 10:78-84.

Besaratinia, A., Pfeifer, G. P. (2003). Weak yet distinct mutagenicity of acrylamide in mammalian cells. Journal of the National Cancer Institute 95:889-896.

Besaratinia, A., Pfeifer, G. P. (2004). Genotoxicity of acrylamide and glycidamide. Journal of the National Cancer Institute 96:1023-1029.

Calcabrini, A., Garcia-Martinez, J. M., Gonzalez, L. et al. (2006). Inhibition of proliferation and induction of apoptosis in human breast cancer cells by lauryl gallate. Carcinogenesis 27:1699-712.

Calleman, C.J., Wu, Y., Tian, G. et al. (1994). Relationships between biomarkers of exposure and neurological effects in a group of workers exposed to acrylamide. Toxicology and Applied Pharmacology 126:361-371.

Covarrubias, V. G., Lakhman, S. S., Forrest, A., Relling, M. V., Blanco, J. G. (2006). Higher activity of polymorphic NAD(P)H:quinone oxidoreductase in liver cytosols from blacks compared to whites. Toxicology Letters 164:249-258.

Dick, R. A., Kwak, M. K., Sutter, T. R., Kensler, T. W. (2001). Antioxidative function and substrate specificity of NAD(P)H-dependent alkenal/one oxidoreductase. A new role for leukotriene B4 12-hydroxydehydrogenase/15-oxoprostaglandin 13-reductase. Journal of Biological Chemistry 276:40803-4810.

Doerge, D. R., Gamboa da Costa, G., McDaniel, L. P., Churchwell, M. I., Twaddle, N. C., Beland, F. A. (2005). DNA adducts derived from administration of acrylamide and glycidamide to mice and rats. Mutation Research 580:131-141.

Doerge, D. R., Young, J. F., McDaniel, L. P. et al. (2005). Toxicokinetics of acrylamide and glycidamide in B6C3F1 mice. Toxicology and Applied Pharmacology 202:258-267.

Ducker, C. E., Stettler, E. M., French, K. J., Upson, J. J., Smith, C. D. (2004). Huntingtin interacting protein 14 is an oncogenic human protein: palmitoyl acetyltransferase. Oncogene 23:9230-9237.

Dybing, E., Sanner, T. (2003). Risk assessment of acrylamide in foods. Toxicological Sciences 75:7-15.

Dybing, E., Farmer, P. B., Andersen, M., et al. (2005). Human exposure and internal dose assessments of acrylamide in food. Food and Chemical Toxicology 43:365-410.

Erdreich, L. S., Friedman, M. A. (2004). Epidemiologic evidence for assessing the carcinogenicity of acrylamide. Regulatory Toxicology and Pharmacology 39:150-157.

Friedman, M. (2003). Chemistry, Biochemistry, and Safety of acrylamide. Journal of Agricultural and Food Chemistry 51:4504-4526.

Friedman, M. A., Dulak, L. H., Stedham, M. A. (1995). A lifetime oncogenicity study in rats with acrylamide. Fundamental and Applied Toxicology 27:95-105.

Fuhr, U., Boettcher, M. I., Kinzig-Schippers, M., et al. (2006). Toxicokinetics of acrylamide in humans after ingestion of a defined dose in a test meal to improve risk assessment for acrylamide carcinogenicity. Cancer Epidemiology, Biomarkers and Prevention 15:266-271.

Gamboa da Costa, G., Churchwell, M. I., Hamilton, P. et al. (2003). DNA adduct formation from acrylamide via conversion to glycidamide in adult and neonatal mice. Chemical Research in Toxicology 16:1328-1337.

Hashimoto, K., Tanii, H. (1985). Mutagenicity of acrylamide and its analogues in Salmonella typhimurium. Mutation Research 158:129-133.

Hassa, P. O., Covic, M., Hasan, S., Imhof, R., Hottiger, M. O. (2001). The enzymatic and DNA binding activity of PARP-1 are not required for NF-kappa B coactivator function. The Journal of Biological Chemistry 276: 45588-97.

Hernandez-Vargas, H., Ballestar, E., Carmona-Saez, P. et al. (2006). Transcriptional profiling of MCF7 breast cancer cells in response to 5-fluorouracil: relationship with cell cycle changes and apoptosis, and identification of novel targets of p53. International Journal of Cancer 119:1164-1175.

Huang, Y., Dai, Z., Barbacioru, C., Sadee, W. (2005). Cystine-glutamate transporter SLC7A11 in cancer chemosensitivity and chemoresistance. Cancer Research 65:7446-7454.

Karin, M. (2006). Nuclear factor-κB in cancer development and progression. Nature 441:431-436.

Katoh, M., Katoh, M. (2004). Identification and characterization of human FHOD3 gene in silico. International Journal of Molecular Medicine 13:615-620.

Katsuoka, F., Motohashi, H., Ishii, T., Aburatani, H., Engel, J. D., Yamamoto, M. (2005). Genetic evidence that small maf proteins are essential for the activation of antioxidant response element-dependent genes. Molecular and Cellular Biology 25:8044-8051.

Konings, E. J. M., Baars, A. J., van Klaveren, J. D. et al. (2003). Acrylamide exposure from foods of the Dutch population and an assessment of the consequent risks. Food and Chemical Toxicology 41:1569-1579.

Lee, J. I., Kang, J., Stipanuk, M. H. (2006). Differential regulation of glutamate-cysteine ligase subunit expression and increased holoenzyme formation in response to cysteine deprivation. The Biochemical Journal 393:181-190.

Lin, S. Y., Cui, H., Yusta, B., Belsham, D. D. (2004). IGF-I signaling prevents dehydroepiandrosterone (DHEA)-induced apoptosis in hypothalamic neurons. Molecular and Cellular Endocrinology 214:127-135.

Livak, K. J., Schmittgen, T. D. (2001). Analysis of relative gene expression data using real-time quantitative PCR and the 2(-Delta Delta C(T)) Method. Methods 25:402-408.

Manière, I., Godard, T., Doerge, D. R. et al. (2005). DNA damage and DNA adduct formation in rat tissues following oral administration of acrylamide. Mutation Research 580:119-129.

Manjanatha, M. G., Aidoo, A., Shelton, S. D. et al. (2006). Genotoxicity of acrylamide and its metabolite glycidamide administered in drinking water to male and female big blue mice. Environmental and Molecular Mutagenesis 47:6-17.

Marsh, G. M., Lucas, L. J., Youk, A. O., Shall, L. C. (1999). Mortality patterns among workers exposed to acrylamide: 1994 follow up. Occupational and Environmental Medicine 56:181-90.

McPherson, J. P., Lemmers, B., Chahwan, R. et al. (2004). Involvement of mammalian Mus81 in genome integrity and tumor suppression. Science 304:1822-1826.

Meunier, V., Bourrie, M., Berger, Y., Fabre, G. (1995). The human intestinal epithelial cell line Caco-2; pharmacological and pharmacokinetic applications. Cell Biology and Toxicology 11:187-194.

Mottram, D. S., Wedzicha, B. L., Dodson, A. T. (2002). Food chemistry: acrylamide is formed in the Maillard reaction. Nature 419:448-449.

Mucci, L. A., Dickman, P. W., Steineck, G., Adami, H.-O., Augustsson, K. (2003). Dietary acrylamide and cancer of the large bowel, kidney, and bladder: Absence of an association in a population-based study in Sweden. British Journal of Cancer 88;84.89.

Neuss, M., Monticone, R., Lundberg, M. S., Chesley, A. T., Fleck, E., Crow, M. T. (2001). The apoptotic regulatory protein ARC (apoptosis repressor with caspase recruitment domain) prevents oxidant stress-mediated cell death by preserving mitochondrial function. Journal of Biological Chemistry 276:33915-33922.

Odlund, I., Romert, L., Clemedson, C., Walum, E. (1994). Glutathione content, glutathione transferase activity and lipid peroxidation in acrylamide-treated neuroblastoma NIE 115 cells. Toxicology in Vitro 8:263-267.

Paulsson, B., Kotova, N., Grawe, J. et al. (2003). Induction of micronuclei in mouse and rat by glycidamide, genotoxic metabolite of acrylamide. Mutation Research 535:15-24.

Pelucchi, C., Galeone, C., Levi, F., et al. (2006). Dietary acrylamide in human cancer. International Journal of Cancer 118:467-471.

Puppel, N., Tjaden, Z., Füller, F., Marko, D. (2005). DNA strand breaking capacity of acrylamide and glycidamide in mammalian cells. Mutation Research 580:71-80.

Ray, R. S., Rana, B., Swami, B. et al. (2006). Vanadium mediated apoptosis and cell cycle arrest in MCF7 cell line. Chemico-biological Interactions 163:239-47.

Rice, J. M. (2005). The carcinogenicity of acrylamide. Mutation Research 580:3-20.

Selvakumar, P., Lakshmikuttyamma, A., Kanthan, R., Kanthan, S. C., Dimmock, J. R., Sharma, R. K. (2004). High exprission of methionine aminopeptidase 2 in human colorectal adenocarcinomas. Clinical Cancer Research 10:2771-2775.

Silvari, V., Haglund, J., Jenssen, D., Golding, B. T., Ehrenberg, L., Tornqvist, T. (2005). Reaction-kinetic parameters of glycidamide as determinants of mutagenic potency. Mutation Research 580:91-101.

Sorgel, F., Weissenbacher, R., Kinzig-Schippers, M. et al. (2002). Acrylamide: increased concentrations in homemade food and first evidence of its variable absorption from food, variable metabolism and placental and breast milk transfer in humans. Chemotherapy 48:267-274.

Stadler, R. H., Blank, I., Varga, N., et al. (2002). Food chemistry: acrylamide from Maillard reaction products. Nature 419:449-450.

Su, L. T., Agapito, M. A., Li, M. et al. (2006). TRPM7 regulates cell adhesion by controlling the calcium-dependent protease calpain. Journal of Biological Chemistry 281:11260-11270.

Subramanian, A., Tamayo, P., Mootha, V. K. et al. (2005). Gene set enrichment analysis: a knowledge-based approach for interpreting genome-wide expression profiles. Proceedings of the National Academy of Sciences of the United States of America 102:15545-15550.

Sumner, S. C., Fennell, T. R., Moore, T. A., Chanas, B., Gonzalez, F., Ghanayem, B. (1999). Role of cytochrome P450 2E1 in the metabolism of acrylamide and acrylonitrile in mice. Chemical Research in Toxicology 12:1110-1116.

Svensson, K., Abramsson, L., Becker, W. et al. (2003). Dietary intake of acrylamide in Sweden. Food and Chemical Toxicology 41:1581-1586.

Tong, G. C., Cornwell, W. K., Means, G. E. (2004). Reactions of acrylamide with glutathione and serum albumin. Toxicology Letters 147:127-131.

Van der Werf, M. J., Pieterse, B., van Luijk, N. et al. (2006). Multivariate analysis of microarray data by principal component discriminant analysis: prioritizing relevant transcripts linked to the degradation of different carbohydrates in Pseudomonas putida S12. Microbiology 152:257-72.

Van Poznak, C., Cross, S. S., Saggese, M. et al. (2006). Expression of osteoprotegerin (OPG), TNF related apoptosis inducing ligand (TRAIL), and receptor activator of nuclear factor κB ligand (RANKL) in human breast tumours. Journal of Clinical Pathology 59:56-63.

Yi, X., Maeda, N. (2005). Endogenous production of lipoic acid is essential for mouse development. Molecular and Cellular Biology 25:8387-8392.

Zhou, Y., Eppenberger-Castori, S., Marx, C. et al. (2006). Activation of nuclear factor-κB (NF-κB) identifies a high-risk subset of hormone-dependent breast cancers. The International Journal of Biochemistry and Cell Biolog 37:1130-1144.

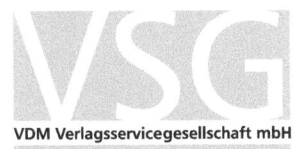

Die VDM Verlagsservicegesellschaft sucht für wissenschaftliche Verlage abgeschlossene und herausragende

Dissertationen, Habilitationen, Diplomarbeiten, Master Theses, Magisterarbeiten usw.

für die kostenlose Publikation als Fachbuch.

Sie verfügen über eine Arbeit, die hohen inhaltlichen und formalen Ansprüchen genügt, und haben Interesse an einer honorarvergüteten Publikation?

Dann senden Sie bitte erste Informationen über sich und Ihre Arbeit per Email an *info@vdm-vsg.de*.

Sie erhalten kurzfristig unser Feedback!

VDM Verlagsservicegesellschaft mbH
Dudweiler Landstr. 99   Telefon +49 681 3720 174
D - 66123 Saarbrücken   Fax   +49 681 3720 1749
www.vdm-vsg.de

Die VDM Verlagsservicegesellschaft mbH vertritt

 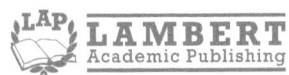 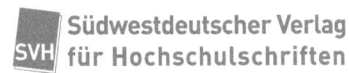

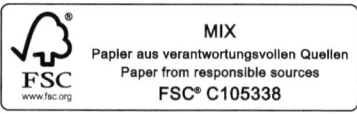

Printed by Books on Demand GmbH, Norderstedt / Germany